TICK-BORNE

Other books by Nora D'Ecclesis...

Mastering Tranquility
Developing Powerful Stress Management Skills

Tranquil Seas
Applying Guided Visualization

Reiki Roundtable

The Retro Budget Prescription
Skillful Personal Planning

I'm So Busy!
Efficient Time Management

Lock Your Door
Passwords, PINS & Hackers

Haiku
Natures Meditation

Adult Coloring
Be a Kid Again!

Equanimity & Gratitude

TICK-BORNE

Questing to Vampire

by

Nora D'Ecclesis

Published by Renaissance Publications, LLC
King of Prussia, PA
ISBN-13: 978-0692867839
ISBN-10: 069286783X

First Edition: April, 2017

TABLE OF CONTENTS

TABLE OF CONTENTS

INTRODUCTION

During a luncheon with my daughter-in-law, the topic of ticks and preventive treatment for the dogs came up in conversation. She and my son have three adorable dogs. Since it was December, I responded with a comment that I start my dog's preventive treatment in March. Danielle then told me a story of a January snow storm years ago and how after digging out she took her dog for a walk on the thin trail made by her shovel because it was so deep. The snow drifts were high but she noticed something tiny walking on the snow, and upon closer examination she said much to her surprise it was a tick – a tick walking on three feet of snow in freezing temperatures probably just waiting patiently for her dog to walk down the path. I knew at that moment my next book would take a look at ticks and tick-borne diseases.

The anecdotal account of repercussions from a tick bite is a good place to start. After one tweet requesting anything people had to say about their experiences with ticks, several hundred people wishing to share emerged on my Twitter messaging. My first interview as it turned out was with a friend who had a most interesting tick-borne story. As I sat in the steak house sitting across from this physician friend who indicated he had a story to tell, I watched the sub-vocalization from his larynx and his frown indicate displeasure. My favorite restaurant might not have been the best choice. There was a slight head twist giving me indication that he didn't like the menu. I asked if he wanted to go someplace else and his verbal response was surprising. He said the steak house was just perfect and he would order the one fish meal on the menu and then tell me his story of the seven years he has endured the horrific effects of his 2010 Lone Star tick bite.

He had excellent recollection of that day, walking his dog and feeling something crawl up his leg. Later that same day he remembered to look and sure enough a tick with a white spot was hanging off his thigh. Using his best surgical skill he carefully removed the tick and its barbed head and cleaned the area with antiseptic. He also watched for a few days and was relieved there was no rash. The first false assumption was that the tick wasn't attached for very long so it was doubtful he would get the dreaded Lyme disease. A few weeks later he even took the precaution of being tested for Lyme disease which was negative. This doctor's anecdotal story began with his passion for hiking thru the wooded areas of the Eastern United States. He described it as meditative and his favorite pastime since moving East from California. He explained that California is devoid of the hardwood forests present all over the eastern United States. Autumn was his favorite time because of the vibrant yellow, orange and red colored leaves and that is when the tick found him.

With a change in facial expressive he indicated and then moved into the core of the discussion which is that the forested areas contain certain dangers that the casual visitor may be completely unaware. It wasn't the bears or bobcats that worried him but rather the insidious creatures of the woods known as ticks, many of which carry a variety of lethal and debilitating diseases. Most of these tick borne diseases have been described over the past few decades and the general public has awareness of the most common, like Lyme disease and Rocky Mountain Spotted Fever.

However, in his case, the clinical changes experienced had not been previously described in the medical literature and were so atypical that the causes of the symptoms were not immediately apparent. The doctor had several episodes of allergic reactions all of which were puzzling as to their origins. He enjoyed a healthy diet from all food groups. The first allergic attack came late at night and he reflected on the potential cause. Since it was 8pm and he had just snacked on pistachio's he assumed that he might be allergic to them and elected to avoid his favorite nuts. The allergic reactions started occurring with greater frequency and the next episode was a little worse after eating French fries. He suspected they might be fried in peanut oil with cross contamination to pistachios.

There were many episodes of allergic reactions including hives and redness that required treatment with antihistamines. Finally one day he found a restaurant that fried everything in olive oil and he enjoyed a hamburger with fries. Many hours later that night, however, he had a severe allergic reaction requiring adrenaline and antihistamines. It was time to see an allergist. He looked to see if the National Institutes of Health might be doing any research on the previously unheard of idea that there could be an allergy to meat that did not emerge until 4-6 hours after ingestion. Therefore, some other antigen was always blamed because typical food allergies are fast to cause rash or even anaphylaxis.

In 2010 the N.I.H. described a "strange beef allergy" occurring after a lone star tick bite, with little information on what to avoid eating. There was no specific treatment. In 2017 there is a laboratory test called Alpha-Galactose IGE Allergy 1,3 clearly indicating the levels of allergic response to beef, pork and lamb. In the words of his doctor his test lit up like a Christmas tree with red positives on all three meats next to normal green negatives on the graph. The laboratory test was done by Quest Diagnostics.

Many ticks are vectors for zoonosis, which are diseases that animals transmit to humans. Several decades ago when I was a child, my father was very ill and in a hospital ICU. The young boy, about my age at the time, who was in the next bed was also very ill from what was described as a wood tick bite. As it turned out the child had Rocky Mountain spotted fever. My relatives were quick to tell me to stay off the wood piles as the family business was construction and there were always wood piles. I learned to check for ticks on my clothing and body daily from the age of ten. My fear of potentially deadly tick diseases was intensified by the death of that youngster who I came to know while visiting my father in the hospital. The ten minutes each day, as I watched them both deteriorate, created lasting memories of their medical conditions. The youngster had such severe rashing on his arms and feet they had to be left exposed so treatment could be constant. In the end the disease was not controllable and he died. My dad passed the following day from heart failure.

In many ways, being aware of the dangers of tick borne illness at such a young age would seem to reduce the potential of a tick borne illness occurring by removing engorged ticks from my body. It did not. They are everywhere I have ever lived or traveled in America. I hike and kayak and play tennis and they crawl up my leg and attach with such routine regularity that I have recently started spraying my shoes before I walk the dog. I am one of the lucky ones having lived in the tri-state areas of New Jersey/New York/Pennsylvania and for a time California, and having never needed treatment for any of the various diseases carried to humans and animals alike by these little critters.

As of April 2017, there are 16 known tick-borne diseases in the USA, several discovered in the last three years. Frequently, a tick will inject more than two pathogens with each bite. *Tick Borne* will identify and define all 16 with more comprehensive explanation of the most common. My intention is to spread awareness of the potential harm of not being treated and to leave the removal techniques, diagnosis and treatment plans to physicians who follow the Centers for Disease Control and Prevention

8

(Atlanta, Georgia) guidelines and National Institutes of Health (Washington, DC) protocols.

If you find an attached tick on your body call your doctor immediately. It is estimated that 300,000 people in the USA alone will have a tick borne disease this year.

I will also take a brief look at tick-borne diseases that harm our companion animals (in the ending pages of this e-book) because our dogs and cats share the horrors of illness from many of the same ticks and the diseases they carry.

The facts presented in this book are for information and awareness purposes only and are not intended to recommend specific courses of treatment or action. Questions about diagnosis and treatment should be referred to a physician or other medical professional.

Tick-borne diseases can be expected to increase in incidence on the short term as people move into new housing developments on the edges of older developments in suburban regions. Extermination of mice – a major intermediate host – might help. Awareness of tick-borne diseases is critical in order to prevent an increase in incidence of the disabling conditions that accompanies them. It is especially incumbent on parents to be aware of these illnesses that ticks can cause and regularly examine children for evidence of ticks and tick bites.

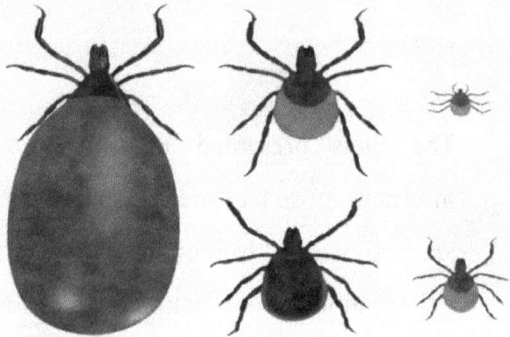

Tick Lifecycle

QUESTING

Questing occurs when a tick senses the body and breath odor from the host animal. They can't fly or jump but they do run quickly toward the highest grass or vegetation and while holding on with their back pair of legs they stretch out their first pair of legs and reach toward the passing person or animal that they plan to feed on. They are the quintessential vampires in the Arachnid Class and questing is the mechanism by which they succeed.

There are hard shell and soft shell ticks with possibly over 1000 species around the world. Their ability to find and attach to the host by questing is a miracle of evolution. It seems they have been doing this for about 145 million years. The proficiency with which they find and feed on a diet of animal blood makes them ecto-parasites but who really cares what they are called when we notice a blood bloated engorged tick sitting on our dog's head?

Questing gets the tick onto the host but finding the perfect spot to dig in for the meal might take a little longer. The tick moves with precision and accuracy up the animal or human to find a soft entrance. With a harpoon or fish hook the barbed hypostome enters the skin, they emit anticoagulant to assure their ability to get the blood they need without the normal process of coagulation preventing them from accomplishing this goal.

The tick usually grows in size until it becomes engorged with blood then drops off and doesn't need to feed again for an extended period. The lifecycle of most ticks includes egg, larva, nymph and adult and as suspected much evidence indicates they simply quest on larger and larger hosts as they get bigger. They are fascinating and if not for the harm they cause would be rather cute little vampires. The problem is that ticks cause tick borne illnesses and carry viruses and bacteria causing fevers, flu like symptoms, paralysis, encephalitis and death. Ticks also cause a relatively newly discovered disease called Alpha-Gal allergy but much more on that later. The latest research also indicates that the female ovaries may contain the pathogens so thousands of the eggs are already diseased before the eggs hatch.

Tick Types and Characteristics

Ticks are arthropods born to females who lay several thousand eggs. The life cycle includes four stages: egg, larva, nymph and adult and is normally completed in a year. They molt between stages, shedding the outer skin. This is the case for both hard and soft shelled ticks. After hatching into the larval tick stage they have only six legs and don't grow the additional two legs until they feed on blood usually from a tiny host they can reach. So, as nymphs and adult ticks they have eight legs with a claw at the end for questing. The legs are segmented and amazing receptors in that the legs have the ability to smell odors, sense temperature changes, feel moisture and sense carbon dioxide levels of warm mammals. As the ticks feed on blood and grow they go higher on the tall grasses to grasp on to larger mammals during questing. Most females breed on the host as adults but have their eggs on the ground.

Ticks found in the United States include…

American Dog Tick (Dermacentor variabilis) is found east of the Rockies and in California. They can cause Rocky Mountain Spotted Fever and Tularemia.

Rocky Mountain Wood Tick (Dermacentor andersoni) is found west of the Rockies. It can cause Rocky Mountain spotted fever, Colorado Tick Fever and Tularemia.

Blacklegged Tick (Ixodes scapularis) is found in northeast, midwest and Texas. It can cause Lyme disease, Anaplasmosis, Babesiosis and Powassan Disease.

Gulf Coast Tick is found on the gulf coast. It can cause Rickettsia parkeri rickettsiosi.

Lone Star Tick (Amblyomma americanum) This is an aggressive tick with an irritating bite that has a sting from the saliva causing irritation. It is found in the northeast, southwest areas of America. It can cause STARI, Tularemia, Erlichiosis and Alpha-Gal Disease Allergy.

Western blacklegged tick (lxodes pacificus) is found in the western US. It can cause Lyme disease and Anaplasmosis.

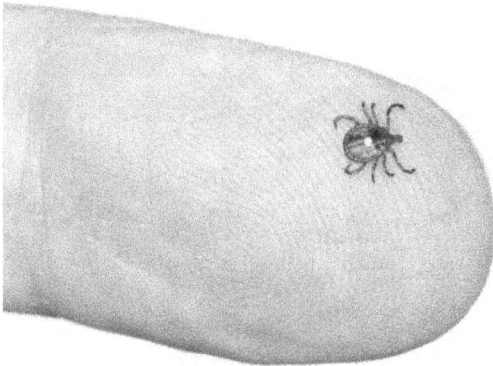

Lone Star Tick

TICK-BORNE DISEASES

Alpha-Gal Allergy 1, 3-galactose

Who doesn't love a barbecue on a summer day? The fun of family and friends, a few beers and juicy steak hot off the grill makes me salivate while writing about it. The picnic that includes a slightly burned hot dog, the Italian sausage with peppers and onions and rare hamburger brings up a visual of the perfect Saturday party outdoors. If we close our eyes we can almost feel the stress free environment created by the barbecue and certainly smell the meat cooking.

There is that one guy off to the side eating salad and chicken wings with what appears to be a voracious appetite. He is the one with Alpha Gal allergy, he is the one who was bitten by a Lone Star tick. That day he pulled out the brownish tick with a white spot altered his life in a way no one anticipated and wasn't even described in the medical literature until 2009 as "strange meat allergy". Using the technique of questing a tick attached itself to this unsuspecting victim and stayed long enough to puncture the skin and inject the Alpha-gal molecule. This could take less than an hour. The end result is that this man will probably never be able to eat red meat again without potential life threatening allergic reaction.

Commins SP, Platts-Mills TA. Delayed anaphylaxis to red meat in patients with IgE specific for galactose alpha-1,3-galactose. Allergy Asthma Res. 2013;13(1):72-77.

The Lone Star tick bite transfers galactose alpha 1,3 galactose from its gut into a victim when it bites a human. The human's immune system then produces an IGE antibody to this sugar in the meat. When the human eats red meat after this process an allergic reaction between the IGE antibody produced by the human's immune system and the alpha Gal sugar in the meat produces the allergic reaction.

The allergic reaction occurs when an IgE antibody reacts with the alpha gal molecule on the meat resulting in a release of histamine and other vasoactive amines which cause damage to capillary walls resulting in leakage of serum in the body tissues including airspaces in lungs and tissue in skin and other organs. Leakage of serum into the lungs may result in actual drowning of the patient in his own body fluid. This is part of anaphylactic shock and will often result in death if not medically treated.

It may seem to the layman that this is an easy problem to fix from a tick bite; it is easy to diagnosis and easy to avoid by simply giving up red meat, but it is not that simple and no one knows at this point if it ever gets better. Remember the physician in our anecdotal has had this for seven years with no change.

Most allergic reactions occur quickly, the bee sting can drop a person in minutes into a life threatening allergic reaction. The child who eats peanuts and gets itchy and has hives can die within minutes. This is not the case with this allergy caused by a tick bite, it is not for 4-8 hours that anyone feels the horrors of the allergic response. Therefore it might take months before the person having this allergy correlates it to the source. Most people look to the last thing they ate and have never read or been told an allergy can take 8 hours to emerge.

Alpha Gal Allergy is a DELAYED 4-6 hours allergic response after eating mammal red meat.

Examples include:

- pork
- beef
- lamb
- venison

- rabbit
- goat
- bison

Or mammal products:

- beef broth
- bacon drippings
- protein powder
- cow's milk
- cheese
- beef gelatins

Or in medical products:

- chemotherapy known as cetuximab
- cardiac pig valves
- beef gelatins used in flu vaccines
- some dental gels

When a person eats mammal meat who has Alpha-Gal antibody the ingested meat causes a histamine release resulting in anaphylaxis. Anaphylactic shock may cause death quickly if not treated by medical personnel. The only way to avoid such a reaction at this time is by avoiding all mammal products which is a great hardship and sometimes difficult task due to lack of information on the ingredients in many products or prepared meals. Fish and poultry are not mammal meats and therefore have not been known to produce the allergy.

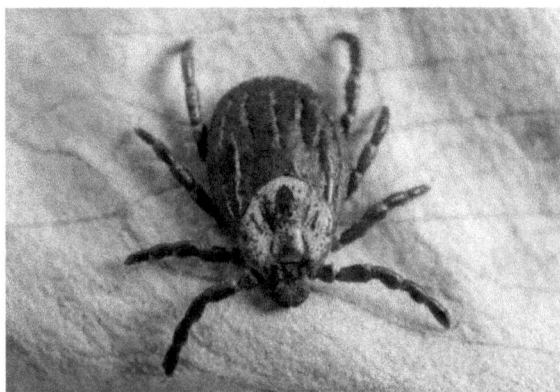

Wood Tick

TICK BORNE BACTERIA

Borrelia Miyamotoi

Borrelia Miyamotoi is a bacteria causing disease from a western black-legged tick seldom presenting with rash but similar in characteristic to Lyme disease but with worse neurological symptoms on occasion. It was found in the 1990's in Japan and is now in America. The standard testing labs for Lyme disease are not effective since it is a different type of bacteria. Antibiotics are used to treat it. This anaerobic spirochete got its first name from a biologist in France named Amedee Borrel. Miyamotoi was named after Kenji Minamoto who discovered it in Japan.

Lyme Disease

Pennsylvania has more cases of Lyme disease than any state in the USA and it is my home.

Last year there were 12,000 documented cases in PA followed closely by New York and New Jersey. It is a dubious distinction to lead the nation in a nasty tick borne illness that in early stages causes flu like symptoms, fatigue, a rash and joint pain and that is if it is caught early. The post Lyme diagnosis, prognosis and treatment plan is far more ominous.

Lyme disease was named after the town of Old Lyme, Connecticut where one of the first concentrations of the disease occurred in the mid-1970s to a group of children with symptoms of arthritis. If you live in the Northeast United States the chances are you probably know someone who has had it. The Centers for Disease Control now acknowledges that there are over 300,000 new cases a year, and many think they are significantly more than that. It is the fastest-growing zoonosis, or animal born disease in North America and Europe.

Ötsi the Neolithic man discovered in the Alps in 2012 probably had Lyme disease. It was found that this 5300-year-old man had the DNA for the bacteria that causes Lyme disease, so it is clearly not a new infection for mankind.

Live Science, 28 Feb 2012, "Ice Mummy May Hold Earliest Evidence of Lyme Disease" by Wynne Parry

Lyme disease is caused by a bacterium named Borrelia Burgdorferi after Willy Burgdorfer who discovered it in 1982. Borrelia is a spirochete, which means it is shaped like a spiral. This is important because of its ability to infect various tissues by burrowing into them. Borrelia's cousin, the world's best-known spirochete, is the one that causes syphilis. Similar to Borrelia, syphilis can affect many different organ systems, and before the advent of antibiotics it was a terrible disease that caused multiple organ failure, dementia and death.

Another important characteristic of borrelia is that it forms what are called biofilms. Biofilms are only beginning to be understood, but they are essentially colonies of bacteria that attach to a substrate and form a sticky, slippery layer. We are all familiar with one common type of biofilm, and that is the plaque on our teeth. We also all know how difficult it can be to get rid of.

In the United States Lyme disease is usually contracted from a deer tick bite, Ioxdes scapularis in the east or the western black leg tick, Ioxdes pacificus, in the west. The Lone Star Tick, Amblyomma americanum which is in the southeast, and is quickly moving up the east coast of the United States, is also a known carrier. Besides Lyme disease, these ticks also carry a host of other bacteria, parasites and viruses which cause problems for people.

The ticks are just one part of a complex and still poorly understood lifecycle of the borrelia bacteria. The main animals involved in this cycle are the white-footed mouse, deer and the occasional human. Recent studies have shown that deer themselves do not harbor a great number of the borrelia bacteria, and attempts to get rid of the deer populations have not been completely successful. This is probably because the main source of the Lyme bacteria is the white-footed mouse and other rodents and even bird populations. It is true however, that because we have removed all their predators, there are many more deer now than there were in the past, and this may be the reason Lyme is so much more common.

Deer ticks live for approximately two years, and have four stages to their lifecycle: egg, larva, nymph and adult, with the last three stages requiring them to obtain a blood meal. Female ticks lay about 2000 eggs each summer. After they have fed, the larva fall off and molt into nymphs and start hunting for their next meal. It is at this nymph stage that Lyme disease is transmitted by the female ticks. It is most commonly transmitted to humans. Tick nymphs are about the size of a sesame seed. The ticks also generally take their second blood meal from rodents or sometimes birds or humans. At this point they can infect their hosts with Borrelia.

After the second meal in early summer they start to molt into adults which are most active in the fall. It's during this adult stage that the ticks attach to deer or dogs, cats, humans and reproduce. The ticks are larger and easier to spot at this point, but can still transmit diseases.

It is during their stage as nymphs when most cases of transmission of Lyme disease to humans occur. There's quite a bit of controversy over how long a tick needs to be attached before it can transmit Lyme and its co-infections. It was generally believed that it took 24 to 48 hours to transmit the disease, but ongoing studies indicate that other factors such as the stage in the lifecycle of the tick, when it had its last meal, and the concentration of the bacteria in the tick are more important factors but much more difficult to predict.

The first symptoms often resemble flu symptoms such as body aches, fever and malaise. You may also develop something called Bell's palsy which is a paralysis of one side of the face. There is also sometimes a rash at the bite site, which resembles a bull's-eye. The percentage of people that develop this rash is an area of great controversy.

Diagnosis includes tests for Lyme with the ELISA and Western blot. Unfortunately, these tests are subject to high numbers of false positives and negatives, which is why they need to be part of a comprehensive clinical diagnosis. If your doctor decides you have Lyme disease he or she will probably prescribe an antibiotic. Because of the lifecycle of the bacteria it is important to take all of the medication to cover all stages in the lifecycle of the bacteria. Luckily, for the majority of people, a single course will be enough to allow them to recover nicely and be fine unless they get another tick bite. The bad news is that having Lyme once does not make you immune to getting it again.

Some people go on to develop Late Stage Lyme or Chronic Lyme, also known as Post-Lyme syndrome. At this point a whole different series of symptoms can arise. One of Lyme's nicknames is the great imitator. This is because Borrelia's ability to attack every organ system can cause patients to have a bewildering group of symptoms that it is difficult to believe are related.

Some of the many symptoms of Late Stage Lyme disease can include arthritis, headaches, fibromyalgia, encephalopathy, fatigue, food and chemical sensitivities, gastrointestinal problems and atrioventricular heart block. Because of Lyme's ability to attack all organ systems this list is extremely long, and patients will often have a mystifying combination of complaints from all parts of their body. This can produce a very debilitating constellation of symptoms that cause Late Stage Lyme patients to be very disabled.

A Lyme disease vaccine is no longer available. The vaccine manufacturer discontinued production in 2002, citing insufficient consumer demand. Protection provided by this vaccine diminishes over time. Therefore, if you received the Lyme disease vaccine before 2002, you are probably no longer protected against Lyme disease.

Prevention

Vigilance is the key here. One way is to try and treat your surrounding areas such as backyards. In some areas in the northeast there are companies that will treat yards with insecticides including leaving cotton balls treated with

Primerithin in tubes for the local mice to build nests with.

When going outside full coverage in light-colored clothes is key. You also should wear socks that can cover your ankles, and that you can tuck your pants into. Clothes you use for walking, running or camping can be sprayed with Primerithine which will last up to two weeks if not washed. Insect sprays containing DEET can be sprayed on the skin to repel ticks. Unfortunately, many Lyme patients develop sensitivities to chemicals and cannot use DEET. However, many tick repellents that use natural essential oils seem to be effective. The biggest focus though still has to be carefully checking yourself, children and pets every day for ticks if you go outside in tick areas. CDC

Several years ago I met an interesting woman who explained she had to stop practicing law due to a severe Lyme disease infection. She told me that back in 1979 she had been a graduate student in archaeology in Arizona, but that summer was offered a position working for a university as an archaeologist on an excavation they were doing in the east. It was late September when they were clearing the site of all brush and debris before starting excavation. She developed a rash on one of her arms. The archaeological was in typical open woodlands. In 1979 Lyme disease was very uncommon. She thought she might have a case of poison ivy, but it didn't itch, and she had never had poison ivy in her life despite spending her youth hiking in the woods. She was busy working on the site, didn't go to a doctor and the rash just eventually went away.

Several weeks later, she was suddenly struck with major asthma problems that seemed to be coming from allergens on the site. Her internist did what was normal in that era, and prescribed steroids. At this point, as you can imagine, she was feeling pretty terrible, but it never occurred to her that it might be related to the rash she had

35

a couple weeks earlier. In retrospect she finally put two and two together, and realized she probably had gotten Lyme disease.

For the next 10 years she basically got on with her life, went back to graduate school, eventually went on to go to law school and had an active busy life. Throughout that time she had constant annoying but not really serious medical issues. These were things like frequent low-grade fevers, swollen glands, body aches and frequent infections. None of her doctors at the time really connected the dots.

She rented a house on a lake but the house had baseboard electric heat. It meant carrying a lot of fire wood in from the outside woodpile. That year was a very mild winter, and one day toward the end of the winter she noticed another rash on her arm where she had been carrying firewood. This time not only did she have a rash, but became quite ill with flulike symptoms. After a few weeks of not getting

36

better, she finally went to see an internist. After listening to her symptoms he suspected that she had Lyme disease. Further testing not only indicated that she had Lyme disease, but he felt that she probably had had it for a long time.

After going through several courses of antibiotics and not really getting any better, she decided to find a Lyme specialist. Despite finding a wonderful Lyme specialist, she entered a difficult period of her life. Over the next 3 to 4 years she did everything she could to regain the life she had been living. She honestly doesn't remember everything she tried, but knows it included several courses of months long IV antibiotics, a 6 month course of homeopathic remedies (herbal remedies). She would improve for a while, but as soon as she stopped the antibiotics she would get worse again.

Eventually, the doctors also diagnosed Babesiosis, which also required treatment. This treatment helped with fevers and the headaches, but again was not a cure. She says that sometimes having Lyme disease and other tick-borne illnesses is like paying a game of whack-a-mole. You manage to get one set of symptoms under control, and a whole new set recur. She said that not only is this beyond annoying, people start to think you are really a lunatic. One week your head hurts, the next week your knees hurt, the next week you can't eat anything because your stomach is so upset. So, even if you find other Lyme disease patients to talk to, they often will have had completely different experiences with the disease. Her biggest problems continue to be neurological and musculoskeletal. These days she primarily takes supportive medications.

Rocky Mountain Spotted Fever

Many years ago my first encounter with Rocky Mountain spotted fever was with the child who I met while I was going to the hospital daily to visit my father. The youngster in the next bed to my dad lived about two weeks from when he was bitten by a tick. He was taken to the hospital in the final stages and the medications were unable to save him. The second time I heard about this disease was from a college professor who found a tick in his groin area upon waking one morning. He removed it according to Center for Disease Control guidelines and saved it in a jar before making a doctors appointment.

Within a week he demonstrated many of the classic symptoms of Rocky Mountain spotted fever with headache, red eye and high fever followed quickly by the distinctive rash. After a skin biopsy and serology he was treated appropriately by his physician and the clinic where he was taken. This story ended well. He recovered with no complications.

Dr. Howard T. Ricketts identified the bacteria causing Rocky Mountain spotted fever.

Unfortunately he later died from a tick borne disease known as typhus which is another rickettsial bacteria. It is interesting and sad that several of the original researchers also died while working to find a cure for Rocky Mountain spotted fever. Drs. McCray and McClintic and their helper, Noguch died during research.

In the early 1920's the governor of Montana lost his daughter and son-in-law to Rocky Mountain spotted fever. He requested and received help from the Federal government to find a cure. They sent Surgeon RR Spenser to help find a way to control or cure this deadly disease. Dr. Spencer did what many researchers did in the early days of research. They used themselves as the experimental case. DR. Spencer pulverized a group of wood ticks and injected it under his skin with some carbolic acid. Much to his joy the vaccine worked. His team of doctors also included Drs. Gettinger, Cowan and Kerlee who did not survive their efforts in the research of Rocky Mountain spotted fever.

This can be a lethal disease and may end in death in a short period of time. He is fully functional a decade later and has no chronic complications. Rocky Mountain spotted fever was first documented in 1896 in Idaho. Many think it was first found in Colorado because the Rockies do run thru many western states including Idaho and Colorado. In 2017 there are 20,000 cases a year normally treated quickly and with excellent results by an alert medical profession with a course of medications that have proven very effective. It is our job to get to the doctor.

Rocky Mountain spotted fever has been the most fatal of the tick borne diseases. It is found in all states of the USA except Hawaii and Alaska. The American dog tick and Brown dog tick and Rocky Mountain wood tick which are all hard bodied ticks as vectors that transmit a gram negative coccobacilus which means long shaped and some round. It is a bacterium that responds well to medical treatment.

Symptoms include:

- fever
- rash
- vomiting
- red eye

RMSF can be transmitted in less than a five hour attachment. It is imperative that once bitten by a tick that medical treatment is obtained immediately. If RMSF is not treated .5% still dies or can get gangrene, hearing loss or need amputations.

Tularemia

The first record of biological aerosolized tularemia bacteria by a tick biting and infecting a host animal used as a vector. Yes, read that sentence again and join me in the knowledge of just how horrific the tick borne diseases can be. Contemplate the ramifications for Tularemia having the potential of biological warfare.

Tularemia is a tick borne bacteria transmitted to humans and rodents causing a skin ulcer at the site of puncture and then swollen lymph nodes. Additionally, there are other forms of transmission and can be lethal if an infected tick bites a rabbit or other rodent that you happen to touch or breathe in the vapors and body parts if a lawn mower shred the animal. In Martha's Vineyard, Massachusetts a person died after mowing a lawn and hitting a rabbit apparently that had been infected by a tick carrying tularemia. This caused an investigation and follow up by the CDC who found other cases around the country with death occurring after lawn mowing body parts becoming aerosolized. It is considered a potential aerosolized biological agent.

As far back as 1715 BC in ancient Canaan Tularemia, called something else, caused an outbreak. Ancient wars probably spread the disease with the help of ticks and some even speculate that the bacteria was intentionally introduced in ancient Anatolia as a form of biological warfare. Experts agree that Tularemia can be aerosolized and requires less than 100 bacteria to be lethal. Trevinsanato, Sirol. (2007) *"The Hittite Plague", an Epidemic of Tularemia and the First Record of Biological Warfare.* Medical Hypotheses, Vol. 69, Issue 6, pp 1371-1374.

Tularemia is named after the California Tulare County where they found the first case in America. G.W. McCoy isolated the bacteria in 1912 while working for the US Public Health. There have been a few documented cases of the disease killing Americans. Three researchers in Boston who were exposed died from it. Recently in Colorado a dozen hikers contracted Tularemia with one death resulting in that state. McCoy GW, Chapin CW. *Bacterium tularense, the cause of plague like diseases of rodents. Public Health Bill* 1912; 53:17-23.

Anaplasmosis

In 2009 David Letterman informed the public he had anaplasmosis from a tick bite contracted while playing with his son near trees. The little vampire ticks are equal in their treatment of anyone who crosses their questing path. They crawl up and bite injecting their bacterias, viruses, protozoa and toxins much of the time. There are of course some ticks that do not carry and diseases.

This nasty bacterium is caused by the bite of a blacklegged tick called Ixodes scapularis found in the northeast and upper midwestern United States. There is also a western blacklegged tick Ixodes pacificus in Northern California. The symptoms of fever, headache, muscle pain, malaise, chills, nausea, abdominal pain, rash and cough make it difficult to diagnose since so many other tick bites have similar symptoms along with things like the flu. Detection may be provided by a Polymerase Chain Reaction test. Microscopic examination of a peripheral blood smear may show micro colonies of anaplasma in white blood cells in about 20% of the patients. Anaplasmosis can be detected by looking for antibodies to the organisms 7-10 days after infection. An indirect immunflorescence assay can be done on serum samples to show and increase in antibody titers by four over a period of 2-4 weeks.

Tick Borne Relapsing Fever

Tick borne relapsing fever is transmitted by "soft ticks" The bite can transmit disease to the human in under twenty minutes. They are not found in tall grass or under wood piles but rather live in a rodent infested den. Some of the rodents they live with include squirrels, chipmunks, mice and prairie dogs that make their homes in old cabins. This of tick makes its way over to one of rodents each night while they are sleeping and since they are "smart" enough to live with such an abundant source of food they only need to feed for a few minutes since one of the rodents is always available. This tick borne illness was unknown to me before writing this book and I must comment that the soft tick is very impressive in setting up home so close to a constant food supply, I have to wonder if they are smarter than the hard ticks but haven't found any way of proving that. The problem comes when people rent old cabins unaware that these ticks are in abundant supply and will also feed on the humans as they sleep. So, if squirrels vacate when a human rents the cabin the ticks "hang out" and continue their lifestyle. The soft tick also live long lives, both the O.hermsitick and B.turicatae tick living 10-20 years.

Dworkin, M.S. et al. *Tick-borne relapsing fever in the northwestern US.* Clinical Infectious Disease 1998; 26:122-31.

In Tick Borne Relapsing Fever, the fever can be as high as 105° F and can include eye pain and headache. It is treatable with antibiotics.

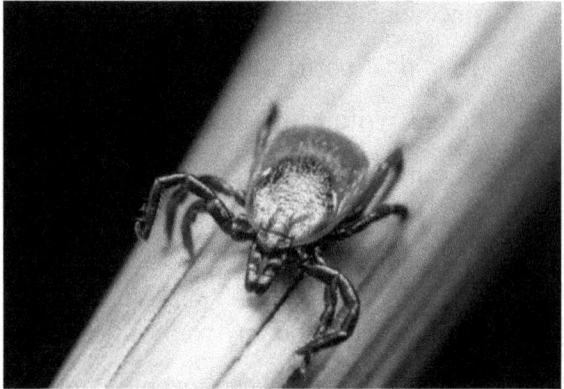

Blacklegged Tick

TICK BORNE VIRUSES

Colorado Tick Fever

There are no medications to treat this tick borne virus. The ticks are found at very high altitudes 8-10,000 above sea level. It is transmitted by the mountain wood tick causing fever, headache, sore throat with gradual improvement followed by a huge relapse, sometimes relapsing into encephalitis and pneumonia depending on the individual's immune system.

Heartland Virus

Heartland Virus is a phlebovirus transmitted by infected blood from a tick. The lone Star tick is the usual culprit. Identification of this virus came three years ago in 2014 in the state of Tennessee. All patients needed hospitalization, there are no specific treatments except support therapy. One of the patients died.

Powassan (POW) Virus

Powassan Virus is a tick borne disease with no vaccines or medications. The symptoms are different from other tick borne illness ranging from seizures, loss of memory and coordination, meningitis to lifelong neurological damage and almost 10% of people who contract it die.

STARI

STARI is an acronym for Southern Tick Associated Rash Illness. The causes of this rash are unknown. The rash measures almost 3 inches after the tick bite and is very red in color. It is caused by the Lone Star tick. It is currently treated in a similar way to Lyme disease. It is also called Masters Disease.

Babesiosis

Babesiosis is the most common co-infection that people get with Lyme disease from a tick bite. Unlike Lyme and several other co-infections, Babesiosis is not a bacterial infection, it is a parasite. One of the most striking aspects of babesiosis is its morphological similarity to malaria. Both are caused by blood borne protozoa that are transmitted to humans by ticks and other insects. In the case of malaria it is by mosquitoes, and babesiosis it is by ticks. They both also have very similar symptoms that again, under the banner of flulike symptoms, including malaise, fever, headache and chills. It also takes a while for the symptoms to develop with an incubation period of up to 8 weeks.

Like Lyme disease this is a disease that needs to be diagnosed by your clinician as the testing for it is not very accurate. It is also easy to confuse with malaria, so a thorough patient history is necessary in diagnosis. For most Lyme patients the diagnosis is made when their symptoms don't resolve after initial antibiotic treatment. This is especially true with continuing fevers and headaches. The treatment for babesiosis is the similar to malaria. The good news is that once you get through the treatment, which may take several courses, most patients feel markedly better especially in terms of fevers and headaches. The prevention for babesiosis is the same as for Lyme or any other tick-borne disease; basically try not to get it in the first place.

New York State Department of Health, *Babesiosis*.

TICK BORNE TOXINS

The pregnant females of the Rocky Mountain Wood Tick, North American Tick and American Dog Tick along with a few others produce a neurotoxin in their salivary gland. At the time the tick bites a human she injects a neurotoxin in her saliva. The horror of this disease is that it seems to prefer children under ten years of age and there is no way at the present time to medicate. The removal of the tick stops the neurotoxin immediately so quick action is needed by the person providing medical care to remove the tick. If the toxin is allowed to remain, the person becomes paralyzed, first in the legs, progressing upward and dies in respiratory failure. Fortunately, this is a rare event.

Dworkin MS, Showmaker PC, Anderson D (1999) *"Tick paralysis: 33 human cases in Washington State, 1946-1996."* Clinical Infectious Disease 29 (6):1435-9.

TICK BORNE DISEASES IN DOGS & CATS

Dogs and cats, cattle and horses, rabbits and rodents are all vulnerable to the devastating tick borne diseases. The ticks can also cause hemolytic anemia and thrombocytopenia (low blood platelets). A rabbit, for example, with several dozen engorged ticks feeding on it will die from the anemia and blood loss. There is a huge loss of livestock from tick borne disease in the United States. The best efforts are barely making a dent but as we have learned the best course is prevention.

Lyme disease or sometimes called Borreliosis from the name of the bacteria, can cause lameness, fever and reduced appetite. The joint pain and advanced symptoms require immediate antibiotic treatment by a veterinarian. There is a vaccine for dogs but not cats. It is transmitted by Deer Tick and Black Legged Tick. Some cases can attack the kidneys (in dogs), causing acute renal failure (known as Lyme Nephritis), the outcome is often fatal. In addition to vaccination, the CAPC recommends year round preventative measures.

Anaplasmosis is carried by deer ticks and western black legged ticks to dogs and cats. They develop joint pain and stomach upset. It is treatable with antibiotics. A big concern is the risk of co-infection (especially with Erlichiosis) and the patient should be tested for both. The animal may present with symptoms similar to Lyme. It is transmitted by the same tick species that carry Lyme.

Tick Paralysis is a toxin and can cause paralysis in dogs in all four limbs. They also have difficulty swallowing and breathing. It is seldom seen in cats. There is an antitoxin that can be administered by a veterinarian.

Rocky Mountain spotted fever is found in the east, midwest and Rocky mountain region. It causes reduced appetite, joint pain, stomach upset in both cats and dogs. They respond well to antibiotics as in humans since it is a bacterial infection.

Ehrlichiosis is transmitted by the Lone Start Tick and is caused by rickettsial. Symptoms include anorexia, bruising and stiffness. It is treatable with antibiotics by a veterinarian. Both Erlichia and Anaplasmosis are transmitted much quicker than Lyme, the tick only needing to be attached 3-4 hours. It is transmitted by several tick species, including Brown Dog Tick.

Tuleraremia is also called rabbit fever. Cats have a terrible prognosis if not treated quickly. They develop high fevers and abscesses near the entrance of the tick bite. There is no vaccine but antibiotics are effective if caught on time.

Babesiosis is a protozoa attacking the red blood cells of both dogs and cats. Dog have a severe reaction including gum infections and dark urine. There is no vaccine and the dog or can carry the protozoa and can relapse. It is transmitted by Brown Dog Tick, but can also be transmitted from dog to dog via bite.

Cyauxzoonosis affects cats that are bitten by the ticks with these protozoa. There is little known about cats and tick borne illness. The best recommendation is year round prevention. This may require indoor confinement for pets that live in high risk areas or who cohabitate with other pets who venture outdoors.

American Canine Hepatozoonosis found in dogs in the southeastern part of the US are infected after eating the tick rather than being bitten by it. It usually results when a dog eats an infected smaller animal. The infection is horrible and frequently kills the dog. Symptoms include high fever and anorexia with muscle wasting. The veterinarian normally treats with antibiotics and anti parasitics but the potential for survival is slim.

Lots of horses are often misdiagnosed for other ailments. They can be afflicted with Lyme and Anaplasmosis, experiencing debilitating lameness, founder (laminitis), edema, eye swelling, and encephalitis. Antibiotics, sometimes long term are used for treatment. Additionally, watch those pretty migratory song birds at our feeders, which usually have ticks who end up in our yard and on our pets, or us.

Routine check-ups by the Veterinarian will help to prevent with excellent forms of treatment and laboratory testing to indicate need for treatment. If an engorged tick is removed from your dog or cat, call the Vet immediately.

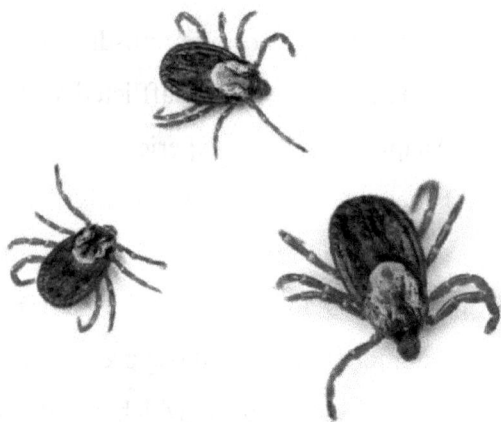

American Dog Tick

CONCLUSION

Awareness of tick-borne diseases in all regions is critical in order to prevent an increase in incidence of the disabling conditions that accompanies them. It is especially incumbent on parents to be aware of these illnesses that ticks can cause and regularly examine children for evidence of ticks and tick bites.

One of the most interesting features of the tick life cycles using the mouse as intermediate host, occurs with the white-footed mouse. Evidence indicates that almost all of the mice tested carry the bacteria for Lyme disease whereas deer only carry it 1% of the time. It would seem that a vaccine to vaccinate the mice with bait boxes as a potential long term solution and is being studied by Richard Ostfeld, a disease ecologist at the Cary Institute of Ecosystem Studies in Millbrook, New York.

The white-footed mouse (Peromyscus leucopus) is being looked at as a potential way to prevent borrelia, which causes Lyme disease. Until an effective human vaccine is available, the next best idea seems to be to explore vaccination of mice using bait boxes so they feed on the vaccine. It does not kill the tick.

The CDC view on vector borne diseases is clear that repellents and tick checks are not enough but the best we have presently to slow the critters down. Tick-borne diseases are far worse internationally than the one described in this book found in The United States. Almost half of the people in the Middle East, Africa and Asia die if a tick transmits Congo hemorrhagic fever to them.

As for me, on any given day summer or winter, my socks are now all white making the little ticks visible as they try to climb up my leg. My ankles and shoes are sprayed with a 30% DEET formula. My clothing and ever present hat is bright colored and treated or sprayed with permethrin. I buy outdoor clothing and shoes pre-treated with permethrin.

A fossil tick was found in New Jersey and after testing indicated it was over 100 million years old. We can safely assume that ticks were here before us and will be around long after we are gone, the best we can hope for is to control the spread of the tick-borne diseases."

Ancient Tick Found In New Jersey Leaves Experts Guessing, Ohio State University 2001."

RESOURCES

columbia-lyme.org/index.html

cdc.gov/lyme/resources/Tickbornediseases.pdf

bayarealyme.org/about-lyme/other-tick-borne-diseases/

cdc.gov/ticks/removing_a_tick.html

niaid.nih.gov/diseases-conditions/tickborne-diseases

epa.gov/insect-repellents/tips-prevent-tick-bites

cdc.gov/ticks/diseases/abroad.html

ncbi.nlm.nih.gov/pmc/articles/PMC3108755/

ars.usda.gov/northeast-area/beltsville-md/beltsville-agricultural-research-center/animal-parasitic-

diseases-laboratory/docs/lyme-disease

johndrullelymefund.org/lyme-disease/

nc.cdc.gov/travel/yellowbook/2016/infectious-diseases-related-to-travel/tickborne-encephalitis

entomology.ucdavis.edu/Faculty/Robert_B_Kimsey/Kimsey_Research/California_Ticks/

capcvet.org

bihint.com

facebook.com/YogaWellnessLauri/

byebyepests.com

ABOUT THE AUTHOR

Nora D'Ecclesis is an American bestselling non-fiction author and poet. Her international #1 bestseller *The Retro Budget Prescription* held the top kindle book downloads in business/self-help for over a year. Nora is a graduate of Kean University of New Jersey with post graduate degrees in administration and education. Her published non-fiction includes Amazon #1 Bestseller *Haiku: Natures Meditation* and books on topics such as time management, personal cyber security password log, guided visualizations, gratitude/equanimity journaling and Zen meditation. Nora's first novel, *Twin Flame* will be published in April, 2017. *Twin Flame* is co-authored by New York Times #1 best-selling author William R. Forstchen.

Nora has a long history of presenting events, retreats and seminars focused on wellness and stress reduction techniques. She enjoys kayaking, hiking and Nordic skiing. Nora lives with her family and wonderful dogs in a suburb of Philadelphia, Pennsylvania.

For more information, please visit

noradecclesis.com